Fast, Lean, Strong:
A Simple Five-Step Guide to Master Intermittent Fasting for Weight Loss, Muscle Gain, and Lasting Health Benefits

KimLien Hoang

Dedicated

*To **everyone willing to start intermittent
fasting (IF) immediately** and **keep IF**
as a routine for a healthier and happier YOU!*

*To **Glen** and **Paddy**, thank you for your love, superb support,
optimism, and always believing in me!*

Acknowledgments

Special thanks

To Jim Edwards for his exceptional guidance and inspiration,
and to Jim's Team for their tremendous support!

To Malgosia and Tina, thank you
for your beautiful friendship
and continuous encouragement!

Contents

Are you still hesitant to jump on the intermittent fasting (IF) bandwagon? Maybe you're unsure if it's the right fit for you, or maybe you're just not quite sure what it entails. Well, let me tell you, IF has been proven time and time again to produce incredible results for those who commit to it. It's time to set aside your doubts and make a decision that will transform your health and your life.

I help Inconsistent Intermittent Fasters become Intermittent Fasting Achievers, so ultimately, by the end of this book, you will have the strategies to:

- Curb your appetite and reduce hunger cravings with the right fasting drinks

- Improve your energy levels and overall well-being

- Boost your metabolism and burn more fat during fasting periods

- Regain control of your eating habits and break through limiting beliefs

- Increase your mental clarity and focus during intermittent fasting

- Enhance your physical performance, endurance, and build your muscle mass

- Strengthen your immune system and overall health with nutrient-dense foods

- Achieve a lean and toned body with exercise while intermittent fasting

- Reach your weight loss goal and maintain a healthy weight

- Establish a sustainable, balanced approach to intermittent fasting for long-term success

Introduction

Plateaus are common in any weight loss or fitness journey, and intermittent fasting (IF) is no exception. Whether you're doing a fast that's 12:12 (12 hours of fasting with absolute no calories, no sugars, no carbs, then 12 hours of eating), 16:8, 18:6, 20:4, or any other variation, you may inevitably hit a plateau at some point. This can be frustrating and discouraging, and it can feel like all our hard work is not paying off. But by adjusting our fasting schedule, such as changing the length of the fasting window, having our exercises more frequently, having our meals with more lean protein and whole fresh foods instead of fried or processed foods, or by incorporating different fasting styles, we can push through the plateau and continue making strides toward our goals. Overcoming these plateaus ensures that we are continually moving toward weight loss and improving our health in the long run rather than feeling stagnant in our progress.

Furthermore, daily exercise is beneficial for breaking through plateaus, helping maintain muscle mass, body lean mass, and preventing the body from adapting to a lower calorie intake. This is important for overall strength, physical health, and a healthy metabolism. In addition to these benefits, consistent exercise can positively impact our cardiovascular health. By having daily physical activity in our routine, we are taking proactive steps toward maintaining a healthy heart and reducing our risk of chronic diseases. Furthermore, we can kickstart our metabolism, burn more calories, and continue toward achieving our health and fitness goals.

Consistency in exercise and intermittent fasting (IF) can lead to a more sustainable, long-term healthy lifestyle. By committing to a regular fasting schedule and daily exercise, we are setting ourselves up for success in the long run. Consistency of doing IF combined with exercise every day is the key to seeing results, and by sticking to a routine, we are more likely to make lasting changes to our health and well-being.

Navigating through the standstills in IF can enhance your body's responsiveness to insulin and help maintain healthy blood sugar levels. Adhering to a regular fasting schedule can positively influence insulin responses, and by moving beyond these standstills, we can keep enjoying these health improvements.

In conclusion, overcoming plateaus in IF and maintaining a daily exercise routine together with whole fresh foods commitment are essential for achieving consistent progress toward weight loss and improved health. We can prevent frustration, maintain a positive mindset, and continue our journey toward a healthier and happier lifestyle by pushing through these plateaus. Remember that progress may not always be linear, and it's expected to experience setbacks. But with dedication, patience, and a positive attitude, we can overcome plateaus and continue toward improved health and well-being to reach our weight and fitness goals.

For all of you who struggle with inconsistency in your IF journey, know that it's never too late to make a change. Even in the midst of stress and overwhelming circumstances, you have the power to take control of your health and well-being. Give your body the excellent care with healthy nutrient-dense food and attention your body deserves with daily exercise. And remember, with discipline, persistence, and the right IF strategies, you can truly achieve incredible health transformation with IF.

So, let's get started!

Chapter 1
Reveal Your Body's True Potential: Mastering the Five-Step Formula for Intermittent Fasting

Intermittent fasting (IF) has gained a lot of attention in recent years for its potential health benefits, including weight loss, improved metabolism, and increased fat burning. However, navigating the world of fasting can be overwhelming, so it's essential you have a clear, step-by-step process to guide you along the way. That's where this book comes in. *Fast, Lean, Strong: A Five-Step Guide to Mastering Intermittent Fasting for Weight Loss, Muscle Gain, and Lasting Health Benefits* is designed to be your comprehensive roadmap to achieving your health and fitness goals through intermittent fasting.

The first step in this process is to **pick the right fasting style that works for you and your body.** We'll guide you through different fasting styles, including 18:6 and alternate-day fasting, and help you experiment to find the schedule that best suits your needs and lifestyle. Once you've found the fasting style that works for you, it's essential to commit to it daily to see actual, sustainable results.

Hydration is key when it comes to fasting and is the focus of our second primary step. We'll show you how to track your water intake and incorporate electrolyte-rich beverages into your routine to ensure you stay adequately hydrated during fasting.

Physical activity is another critical component of a successful intermittent fasting journey, and our third main step will guide you through how to schedule regular workouts, set achievable fitness goals, and track your progress to stay motivated and on track.

Eating the right foods during your eating windows is our fourth main step. We'll help you prioritize nutrient-dense foods, plan and prepare meals ahead of time, and practice mindful eating to ensure you're getting the most out of your eating windows.

Finally, **tracking and analyzing your eating patterns is crucial** for long-term success with intermittent fasting, which is why it's our fifth main step. We'll show you how to keep a food diary, identify triggers for overeating, and adjust your eating patterns based on your observations.

By following the step-by-step process outlined in this book, you'll be equipped with the knowledge and tools to successfully curb appetite, reduce hunger cravings, boost metabolism, burn more fat during fasting periods, reach your ideal weight, and maintain a healthy weight for the long term. Are you ready to embark on this transformative journey?

Your Most Effective Simple Five-Step Intermittent Fasting Overview

1. **Choose the right fasting style** for you and your lifestyle and **commit to doing it** weekly or daily.

2. Track your water intake and incorporate **electrolyte-rich beverages** and **hot teas** into your daily routine.

3. **Schedule daily workouts**, set realistic, achievable fitness goals, and track your progress.

4. **Prioritize whole, nutrient-dense foods**, plan and prepare meals ahead of time, and practice mindful eating.

5. Keep a food diary, **identify triggers for overeating**, and **adjust** your fasting, exercising, and eating patterns **to keep practicing IF persistently every other day and/or every week**.

Let's go!

Chapter 2
Customizing Your Fast: Tailoring a Fasting Schedule that Fits Your Style

This chapter will help you:

- Identify the fasting schedules that align with your daily routine, work schedule, and social commitments

- Understand the importance of consulting with your healthcare professional to determine the best fasting style for your needs

- Experiment with different fasting schedules and pay attention to your body's response to determine the most effective schedules for your needs

- Remember your experiences during the experimentation phase to understand how different fasting schedules impact your body and mind –both successes and struggles

- Use your phone for more effective IF support

By the end of this chapter, you should be able to find the best fasting style and schedule that fits your lifestyle and goals to effectively maximize fasting results.

From Depressed and Isolated to Vibrant And Confident: How I Shed My Weight and Reclaimed My Life

At the age of 41, I found myself facing a mountain of struggles. As a single mom, I had been through many hardships, but the one that seemed impossible was my weight. I had ballooned to a size that I didn't recognize, and it left me feeling unmotivated, depressed, and isolated. I longed to find my old self – vibrant, confident, and full of life. But it seemed like an impossible dream with each passing day.

The turning point came when my best friend announced her bachelorette party. I wanted nothing more than to celebrate with her, but when I tried on all of my dresses, not one fit. I was at size 6 and all the old dresses I have in my closet are size 2. I couldn't afford to buy a new dress at the time, truthfully, but I was determined to make it work, to get my confidence back, and to fit into my most favorite blue dress. I knew I had under two weeks to shed the weight to get back to size 2.

I had already tried countless diets in the past, but none of them had worked for me. Then, I stumbled upon the concept of intermittent fasting. With a deep breath and a resolve to make a change, I decided to try it. I started with a 12:12 fasting style (12 hours of fasting then 12 hours of eating window), then 16:8, 18:6, and eventually 20:4. I coupled this with two planned meals daily and 20 minutes of exercise every other day.

After four days, I felt defeated because not much had changed; I had barely progressed and was ready to throw in the towel. But something inside me urged me to keep going.

On the fifth day, I switched to an entire 18-hour fasting window, consuming only lime-herb electrolyte water and hot herbal tea during the fasting times. I prepared my one meal at family dinner time with my son (I cooked breakfast for him and packed lunches for him to have at school) with only anti-inflammatory and immunity foods. I pushed myself to increase my cardio workouts to 45 minutes daily. I eventually added hour-long sessions on the elliptical into my daily routine on day seven.

Somehow, I did not feel starved at all during my fasting times. The electrolyte water and slowly sipping the hot herbal tea blend really helped. It was great when I had a clear goal and stuck to it. I focused on my goal and did my best to achieve it, ultimately ignoring what might interfere.

The result was nothing short of miraculous. I could hardly believe the transformation I was experiencing. In less than two weeks, I had shed the weight burdening me, fitting into my favorite blue dress with ease. But it was not just the weight loss; I felt great in my whole body, had regained my confidence, and perhaps even regained what people often call a lost soul.

Standing in front of the mirror in my blue dress, I felt a surge of pride and joy. I was reclaiming my body, confidence, and sense of self.

My friend's bachelorette party was a night to remember. I danced, laughed, and shared in the love and happiness of my best friend. I felt and looked amazing, and I truly felt light for the first time in many years. As I recounted my journey to my best friend, she was so happy at my transformation. And in that moment, I knew that I had emerged victorious.

My experience with intermittent fasting was real life-changing. I discovered a new sense of energy, vitality, and health. I felt less fatigue, gained muscle mass with the right foods and daily exercise, and my weight decreased so significantly. I realized that with **the right approach to intermittent fasting that works best for me** coupled with a **steadfast commitment to exercise** and **wholesome, nourishing meals**, change is not only possible but inevitable. After less than a month, I felt like a new person – healthier, happier, and more radiant than I had been in years.

I hope that by sharing my story, others will find the inspiration and motivation to embark on their own journey to health and wellness. Intermittent fasting (IF) may seem daunting at first, but the rewards are immeasurable. IF has transformed my life, and I believe it can do the same for anyone willing to embrace the possibilities of change. So, to anyone who feels trapped in their struggle, remember that transformation is within your reach with determination, perseverance, and the right lifestyle choices. I am a living proof that the human spirit can triumph over any obstacle and that each of us holds the power to rewrite our story.

Possible Tools and Resources You Will Need

Highly recommended books:

1. *Outlive: The Science and Art of Longevity* by Peter Attia MD.

2. *Neurofitness: A Brain Surgeon's Secrets to Boost Performance & Unleash Creativity* by Dr. Rahul Jandial.

3. *Intermittent Fasting Diet Guide + Cookbook* by Dr. Becky Gillaspy.

These books offer insights and practical tips on how the leading trio of whole, nutritious food choices, the right enjoyable exercises, and an excellent intermittent fasting strategy can significantly help improve our health and weight goals, with the important addition of nightly, good-quality sleep, which can help struggling intermittent fasters make informed decisions about their fasting schedules and styles and help them stay on track.

- Consulting with healthcare professionals, such as nutritionists and registered dietitians, is crucial in determining the best fasting style for your own needs (especially if you are currently under a strict diet, take certain medication that requires food, have specific chronic disease, or are pregnant or breastfeeding), ensuring that your health and well-being are prioritized throughout your fasting journey.

- Websites such as WebMD and Mayo Clinic provide valuable information on different fasting styles, their potential effects, and their impact on health and well-being.

So, How Do You Tailor a Fasting Schedule that Fits Your Lifestyle?

Step 1: Write down different fasting schedule variations

Start by checking your work schedules for the month, week, and day, then write down the various intermittent fasting schedules that you can potentially incorporate into your lifestyle weekly to daily. You do need to write these down before picking your schedules so that you can actually follow your IF schedule(s) with commitment.

This includes options such as:

1. The 12:12 method (12 hours of fasting with absolute no calories, no sugars, no carbs, then 12 hours of eating)

2. The 16:8 method (16 hours of fasting then 8 hours of eating)

3. the 18:6 method (18 hours of fasting then 6 hours of eating – highly recommended cause I do this every other day it works well for me)

4. The 20:4 method (20 hours of fasting then 4 hours of eating – again, highly recommended. I do this twice a month)

5. Or intermittent fasting every other day (full 24 hours of fasting and full 24 hours of eating window). <u>Note</u>: More details on the proper nutrition and daily adequate protein amounts for each fasting option coming up in Chapter 5.

Consider the IF hours that work best for your daily routine, your weekly family or personal schedule, your work schedule, and your social commitments.

Different schedules may work better for you on certain days of the week or during specific months of the year.

By mapping out these clear options, you can see which fasting schedules align with your needs the best on your particular days, weeks, and months ahead.

It's very important to write down first, then pick the IF times to <u>mark on your calendar,</u> and <u>follow these IF schedules CLOSELY</u>. Yes, you have to take actions to achieve results, my friends!

Step 2: Consult with your healthcare professional

If you're taking medication that requires you to eat at certain times, breastfeeding, on a strict diet, or if you have a history of eating disorders, it's crucial to consult with your healthcare professional. They can help you determine the best fasting style for your needs, prioritizing your health and well-being throughout your fasting journey.

Step 3: Experiment with different fasting schedules

Once you've mapped out the various fasting schedules and consulted with your healthcare professional, it's time to experiment. Try different fasting schedules and pay attention to your body's response. Keep track of how you feel physically and emotionally during each fasting window. For example, you may find that after experimenting with the 16:8, 18:6, and 20:4 schedules, the latter two fasting styles work best for you. You can determine the most effective schedules for your needs by narrowing down your options.

Step 4: Keep a journal, either physically or on your phone

It's important to keep a journal of your experiences during your experimentation phase. This can be a physical journal or simply notes on your phone. Document your progress, how you feel during fasting periods, and any difficulties you may face. This journal will serve as a valuable tool in understanding how different fasting schedules impact your body and mind.

Step 5: Schedule your fasting hours, fasting drink times, and specific planned meals on your phone

This is very important because your phone is your valuable ally in helping you stay on track with your fasting routine. By using your phone's alarm and reminder features best, you can set yourself up for success and make the most of your intermittent fasting journey.

1. **Set reminders or alarms on your phone that prompt you to drink water.** Reminder: stick with drinking three one-liter water bottles a day, high-quality herbal teas, or black coffee. Staying hydrated not only helps you feel better during fasting but can also help minimize hunger pangs and support overall health. By using your phone to remind you to drink regularly, you can ensure that your hydration stays on track throughout the day.

2. **Set a reminder on your phone to help you stay committed to your daily exercise** goals: going for a walk, doing yoga, jogging, running, getting on your elliptical at home, jumping jacks, or hitting the gym.

3. **Establish a set eating window and use alarms to signal the start and end**

of this window to help you structure your meals and ensure you get quality nutrients from fresh, nutrient-dense, whole foods. **By setting reminders on your phone for those quality meal times**, you can actively plan ahead and stick with them to support your body's needs and make the most of your eating window.

Add inspirational quotes or affirmations as daily reminders on your phone to provide extra motivational boosts.

Keep the below tips in mind to plan your fasting schedule ahead of time.

Nine Simple Yet Effective Ways to Beat Sugar Cravings, Calorie Temptations, and Exercise Struggles in Intermittent Fasting

1. **Stay hydrated:** Sometimes, we mistake thirst for hunger, which leads to unnecessary snacking. Drink plenty of water daily to stay hydrated and ward off cravings.

2. **Plan balanced meals during your eating hours:** Ensure your meals include a good balance of lean protein, healthy fats from natural fresh foods, fresh fruits and veggies, and fiber-rich carbohydrates to keep you satiated and prevent sugar cravings and empty calories in the next fasting window timeframe.

3. **Incorporate more nutrient-dense foods:** Focus on including nutrient-dense foods like fresh vegetables and fruits, lean proteins, and whole grains in your meals during your eating windows to ensure that you are getting the essential nutrients your body needs, which can reduce cravings for unhealthy foods during your fasting times.

4. **Practice mindful eating:** Slow down and savor your meals. Pay attention to your body's hunger and fullness cues to prevent overeating during your eating windows and keep cravings at bay.

5. **Have high-quality drinks** such as premium herbal tea with natural sweetness and alkaline water with high pH readily available to satisfy your cravings without derailing your fasting goals.

6. **Find alternative ways to cope with stress:** Stress can often trigger cravings for sugary and calorie-dense foods. Practice stress-reducing activities such as meditation, yoga, or deep breathing to manage stress without turning to food.

7. **Schedule regular exercise:** Incorporating daily exercise activities that you

enjoy doing into your routine can help you regulate your appetite, drink more water, reduce cravings, and boost your mood, making it easier to adhere to your intermittent fasting plan.

8. **Avoid processed foods at all costs:** Processed foods are often high in sugar and unhealthy fats and lack in essential nutrients. Opt for whole, unprocessed foods to support your health during your eating windows.

9. **Seek support:** Join a support group, find a fasting buddy, or seek guidance from a nutritionist or healthcare professional to stay motivated and accountable in managing your cravings, maintaining a healthy diet, and adhering to an intermittent fasting regimen.

10. **Keep a detailed journal.** To start, keeping a detailed journal of your fasting style, including the duration and timing of your fasting windows with your fasting drinks on your physical notebook or your phone notes, is essential.

Example:

KimLien's	Monday	Tuesday	Wed	Thurs
Fasting Hours	10 PM Sun to 6 PM Mon	10 PM Mon to noon Tue		
Fasting Drinks (alternate those drinks every hour or two)	Hot herbal teas, alkaline water with fresh mint or fresh herbs, black coffee, hot teas, water with apple cider vinegar (optional)	Hot herbal teas, alkaline water with fresh mint or fresh herbs, black coffee, water, wot teas, water with apple cider vinegar (optional),		
Exercise	30 minutes elliptical + 6x30 jumping jacks	30 minutes elliptical + 6x50 aerobic step jumps		
Post-Fasting Meal Time(s)	Wild salmon fillet + green beans + quinoa	Steak fillet or chicken breast + mushrooms + sweet potatoes		
Repeat				

Tip: Copy and paste the schedule every Sunday, adjust if there're changes, so you can start the new week solid and consistent.

This will help you identify the best fasting schedule that aligns with your lifestyle and allows you to stick with it consistently.

Record any cravings or mood changes to identify patterns related to your eating habits.

Also, track the drinks you consume during fasting, as some beverages can impact your fasting state. For example, some people find that black coffee or herbal tea helps curb their appetite during fasting, while others prefer plain water or a combination.

For me, drinking hot green tea, white tea, and certain herbal tea blends in the morning and during fasting won't cause tummy upset, but black coffee does, even when I add some cream.

In addition, I can drink way more alkaline water, or lemon and lime water with fresh herbs of mint, basil, and rosemary than just plain tap or filtered water.

When it comes to breaking your fast, keeping a record of what you eat during your eating windows and how it makes you feel can help pinpoint which foods make you feel satisfied and energized and which leave you feeling sluggish or craving more. Remember that your food portion size during your eating times contributes to achieving your health and weight goals.

Adjust your living space, office, kitchen, and living room to minimize exposure to food during fasting periods, keeping snacks out of sight.

Checklist for Your Action Steps

- ✓ <u>Pick specific fasting hours</u> that work best for you, your work, and your family time so you can <u>stick to them without interruption</u>.

- ✓ <u>Mark the fasting timeframe and exercise time on your calendar</u> and set a <u>reminder on your phone</u> for each day before and during fasting hours.

- ✓ <u>Set specific fasting drink times at specific hours for each day on your phone</u> according to your work, commute, and family times for that particular day.

- ✓ <u>Set up specific meal plans with lean protein and whole food fresh nutrition</u> for <u>each meal of each fasting day</u>.

- ✓ <u>Clear your pantry, fridge, and counter areas of snacks, foods, and drinks</u> that might make you break your fasting.

- ✓ <u>Let your family members, friends, and/or co-workers know</u> (if you're comfortable with them) and/or join IF groups so they can support you.

- ✓ <u>Commit to your fasting goals and do your best not to break your fasting hours</u>. If you must break your IF hours earlier or can't do it on the day you're marked for, <u>start your fasting hours again the next day</u>.

Chapter 3
Crush Cravings with Hydration:
The Key to Successful Intermittent Fasting

Welcome to Chapter 3!

In this chapter, we will discuss **the importance of staying hydrated** during your intermittent fasting journey. **Hydration is key** to supporting your body's functions during fasting periods, and it can also help you **curb cravings** and **reduce hunger**. We'll review some simple ways to ensure you're getting enough fluids throughout the day to support your fasting goals.

This chapter will help you:

- Understand the importance of staying hydrated during intermittent fasting to support your body's functions and fasting goals.

- Set a specific goal for your daily water intake and track your progress to ensure you're staying hydrated.

- Incorporate electrolyte-rich beverages like herbal teas and coconut water to replenish electrolytes and add variety to your fluid intake during fasting periods.

- Develop strategies to ensure easy access to hydration throughout the day, even when you're on the go.

- Recognize signs of dehydration and adjust your water intake to stay hydrated during fasting periods.

The Surprising Drink that Helped Me Beat Sugar and Carb Cravings During Intermittent Fasting

Back to my story of trying to lose weight with IF in Chapter 2.

The first few days were a real struggle for me. I broke my fast with milky coffees and carb-loaded pastries like my favorite croissants, unable to resist my cravings. I felt defeated, isolated, and disappointed in myself. I knew I needed to find a way to stick to my fasting plan without giving in to temptation.

So, after I stopped buying croissants and cleared other carb-loaded foods and snacks away, I researched, devoured books, and studied the most effective and natural drinks to consume during fasting. After much consideration, I decided to commit to only hot herbal teas and electrolyte waters with or without fresh mints or herbs to sustain me through my fasting hours.

I'm a big coffee fan, too, but having black coffee on an empty stomach just doesn't work for me, and even though cream (no sugar) can be added to black coffee, I just don't enjoy the taste.

So, initially, it was a very difficult adjustment, but I was determined to make it work.

As the days passed, I found strength in my determination. By day 5, I had already lost almost 4 pounds; by the end of day 11, I had shed over 9 pounds. More importantly, I felt a renewed energy and focus I hadn't experienced in years. I no longer needed to rely on naps to get me through the day.

The changes I experienced were profound. I transformed my life by taking concrete actions to stop breaking my fast and instead embracing fasting drinks that were both enjoyable and effective. I had proven that I had the power to change and that change was within my reach.

Reflecting on my fasting journey, I realized that fasting without strategies and determination often increases cravings. If I wanted to achieve my health and weight goals, I had to do something different. I couldn't expect my health to fix itself and my weight not to drop. It was up to me to take action and NOT give up.

I had found a new sense of purpose and control over my health. My story served as a reminder that, with determination and the right drinks we enjoy, we can overcome our cravings and obstacles, achieve our fasting, health, and weight goals, and experience a transformation beyond the physical. I am proof that it is never too late to improve your life.

Possible Tools and Resources You Will Need

- Water-tracking apps like MyFitnessPal and WaterMinder can help you monitor daily water intake and stay on track with your hydration goals.

- Marked electrolyte water bottles (just my own old-fashioned way, I **marked 1, 2, 3** for my three one-liter water bottles for my daily drinks) can make tracking your fluid intake easy and ensure you get enough fluids throughout the day.

- Various green, white, and herbal tea blends – this is important because these hot teas can add variety to your fluid intake and provide additional health benefits during fasting periods – **more on these and why in Step 3 below.**

- Hydration-reminder apps like Drink Water Reminder and Hydro Coach can send you regular reminders to drink water throughout the day and help you stay on top of your hydration goals.

Step 1: Set a goal to drink at least two to three one-liter water bottles per day in addition to hot tea

Setting a clear goal for your daily water intake can help keep you accountable and ensure you're getting enough fluids to support your fasting efforts. Aim to drink at least two to three one-liter water bottles throughout the day in addition to hot tea. This will help ensure you stay hydrated and will support your body's fasting functions.

For example, you can start your day by drinking a full one-liter water bottle in the morning then aim to finish another one-liter bottle by mid-afternoon and another before and after dinner.

By setting specific goals for your water intake, you can track your progress and ensure you're staying on track throughout the day.

Step 2: Mark water bottles for easier tracking of daily water intake to stay accountable

To make tracking your daily water intake easier, consider marking your water bottles to indicate how much you should drink by specific times of the day. This visual reminder can help you stay accountable and ensure you get enough fluids to support your fasting goals.

For instance, you can mark the numbers on the side of the water bottle to indicate the number of water bottles you are drinking or have finished. This can help you stay on track and meet your daily hydration goals.

Step 3: Incorporate electrolyte-rich beverages like hot herbal teas or coconut water

In addition to plain water, incorporating electrolyte-rich beverages like hot herbal teas or coconut water can help support your hydration needs during fasting periods. These beverages can help replenish electrolytes and minerals lost during fasting and add some variety to your fluid intake throughout the day.

For example, you can enjoy a cup of hot black, green, or white tea in the morning since those teas have some caffeine, and hot herbal teas in the afternoon to help keep you hydrated and support your fasting efforts.

Why Hot Tea?

Hot tea is an essential beverage, especially during long fasting hours, as it helps you sip slowly and extends your liquid intake over a longer time. Staying hydrated is essential when fasting, and hot tea is the perfect solution. Sipping hot tea supports your body's hydration needs and stops you from feeling overly thirsty during extended fasting periods.

Furthermore, high-quality herbal teas have natural sweetness, which can help eliminate the distraction of sugar and carb cravings. Instead of reaching for unhealthy snacks, a delicious and satisfying cup of hot tea can provide a comforting alternative. With so many varieties and flavors, you can find the perfect hot tea to enjoy during fasting.

In addition to helping with hydration and curbing cravings, specific herbal teas can offer unique health benefits that water alone doesn't provide. The array of nutrients and antioxidants in green and white teas and many herbals can be an excellent healthy addition to your fasting routine. So, the next time you need a warm, comforting beverage, consider reaching for a hot cup of tea and reap the many health benefits it offers.

Always aim for <u>zero-added sugar</u> on ALL food and drink labels when you shop.

Step 4: Keep your hot herbal tea and one-liter water bottle with you at all times during your IF hours to ensure easy access to hydration

To ensure you're getting enough fluids throughout the day, always keep a cup of hot herbal tea and your one-liter water bottle with you. This ensures that you have easy access to hydration and can take regular sips of water or tea throughout the day.

For instance, you can carry a reusable water bottle wherever you go and keep a thermos or insulated cup for your hot herbal teas. This makes it easy to stay hydrated and support your fasting goals, even on the go.

Step 5: Pay attention to signs of dehydration and adjust your water intake as needed

Finally, pay attention to signs of dehydration and adjust your water intake as needed. If you experience symptoms like dry mouth, headache, or dizziness, it could be a sign that you need to add some electrolyte-rich beverages to help replenish your fluids and support your body's functions.

By implementing these strategies and using these tools, you can get enough fluids to support your body's functions and stay adequately hydrated during intermittent fasting. This will not only help you curb cravings and reduce hunger but also maintain overall health and well-being on your fasting journey.

Congratulations on completing Chapter 3!

Keep up the great work, and we'll see you in the next chapter as we explore the keys to successful intermittent fasting.

Checklist for Your Action Steps

- ✓ Pick healthy fasting drinks and commit to only having those during your intermittent fasting hours to stay hydrated and support your body's functions and fasting goals.

- ✓ Mark your water bottles to set a specific goal for your daily water intake: at least three liters of electrolyte water and two to three cups of hot tea every day .

- ✓ Track your fasting drink intake progress to ensure you're hitting your daily goals and staying hydrated.

- ✓ Take the drinks with you even when you're on the go to ensure easy access to hydration throughout the day and to crush your sugar or food cravings.

- ✓ Recognize any signs of dehydration and quickly adjust your water intake accordingly.

Chapter 4
Move More, Flexing Fasts: Building Muscle and Burning Fat through Exercise

In this chapter, we will discuss how to schedule regular workout sessions to make exercise a consistent part of your routine, incorporate a mix of cardio and strength training exercises, set achievable fitness goals, find a workout buddy or join a fitness class, and gradually increase the intensity and duration of your workouts as your fitness level improves.

This chapter will help you:

- Understand the importance of <u>scheduling regular workout sessions</u> to make exercise <u>a consistent routine.</u>

- Incorporate a mix of cardio and strength training exercises into your routine to <u>maximize the benefits</u> for your <u>metabolism and weight-loss</u> goals.

- <u>Set achievable fitness goals to keep you motivated</u> and focused on increasing physical activity.

- Understand the benefits of finding a workout buddy or joining a fitness class to stay accountable and motivated to exercise regularly.

- <u>Gradually increase the intensity and duration of your workouts</u> to continue challenging your body and <u>see improvement.</u>

The Daily Routine that Saved Me: Overcoming Arthritis and Weight Struggles

I want to share my journey of overcoming obstacles, personal growth, and the triumph of the human spirit. As I shared my story in Chapter 2 about my friend's bachelorette party and blue dress. At this same time frame, in addition to the weight gain, I also found myself struggling with terrible neck pain for a long, long time. I knew I was desperate for both: get rid of the neck pain and the weight together, and I was determined to make it happen.

I decided to practice intermittent fasting daily, with the ultimate goal of shedding the extra weight and somehow get rid of the persistent pain. However, my plans were quickly met with a roadblock: my doctor informed me that I needed to stay focused on solving the neck pain first, and I needed to see a physical therapist twice a week because I had arthritis in my C3-4, causing severe nerve impingement on the right side of my upper body. This news was disheartening, and to make matters worse, the cost of physical therapy, even with my health insurance, was proving to be a financial burden.

As I grappled with the stress and overwhelm of balancing work, driving, therapist appointments, dropping and picking my son up after work, and cooking, it became clear that I had more stress than ever with no time for myself at all. I knew I had to make a change to find time for myself and address my health and weight goals.

I decided to take matters into my own hands and find a way to exercise within my limited time.

My supportive boyfriend helped me purchase a used elliptical (sensing my serious determination :-)), and I got a very inexpensive shallow plastic aerobic step jump and some resistance bands from Amazon.

These simple tools allowed me to begin incorporating exercise into my daily routines. I started mornings by getting on the elliptical with my empty tummy before showering and heading to work. Throughout the day, I made a point of jumping on the aerobic step during any free moment. I utilized the resistance bands to stretch my shoulders to help relieve the neck pain and do jumping jacks in my office or, basically, in most rooms at home whenever I need an energy boost for the day.

As I settled into this new routine, I saw powerful changes in my body and mindset. I realized that combining daily exercise and fasting was the powerful catalyst I needed to transform my health. Not only was I shedding the extra weight (with IF hours and nutritious meals with lean protein) and gaining muscle mass (with my daily exercises), but I was also finding relief from the chronic neck pain that had been weighing me down.

Through this journey, I learned that <u>fasting without exercise and excellent nutritious food choices with the right amount of lean protein</u> (which I will talk more about in the next chapter) <u>is not as effective</u> and <u>could cause bone and muscle mass loss</u>. The **daily commitment to exercise truly made the difference**, allowing me to boost my health, maintain and build my muscle mass, and ultimately achieve both get rid of my neck pain and my ideal weight goal.

Today, I stand as living proof that change is possible and that we can transform our lives with resilience, determination, and the power of daily exercise. I hope my story can inspire anyone facing their own obstacles and that they, too, can find the strength within themselves to overcome and thrive.

Possible Tools, Apps, and Resources You Will Need

- Fitness apps like Nike Training Club, Runkeeper, and Strava can help track and plan your workouts, ensuring you stay consistent with your exercise routine

- Elliptical or indoor bike at home (you can get a used one on local Facebook Marketplace, Amazon, or other marketplaces quickly)

- Aerobic step jumps – both for in-office and/or at-home

- Resistance bands

- Dumbbells or kettlebells

- A fitness tracker or smartwatch can monitor your progress and keep you motivated to reach your fitness goals

- A workout planner or journal can help you schedule and track your workouts, keeping you organized

- Online workout videos or classes can provide guidance and structure to your workouts and offer variety and new challenges to keep your routine fresh and engaging.

Daily Exercises with No Required Equipment:

- Jumping jacks and squats anytime, anywhere, for convenient strength training exercises to strengthen muscles and boost metabolism.

- Do jumping jacks and squats as long as you comfortably can, ideally 30 to 60 jumping jacks each time, then switch to 20–30 squats at a time for 4 to 6 times daily.

So, let's talk about scheduling your regular workout sessions.

Mark and highlight specific days and times on your calendar or set a schedule and reminder on your phone for exercise; yes, seriously, just like you would for any other important appointment. By doing this, you are **making exercise a priority** and **ensuring** that it becomes **a regular habit**. This consistency will help you stay committed to your fitness goals.

First, it's important to incorporate a mix of cardio and strength training exercises into your routine. Cardio exercises like running, cycling, or dancing (or on elliptical for indoor…) can help improve your cardiovascular health and burn calories. On the other hand, strength training like weightlifting or bodyweight exercises (like doing step jumps for indoor…) can help build muscle and boost your metabolism. By combining these two types of exercises, you maximize the benefits for your metabolism and weight loss goals.

Next, daily exercise helps tone your body and shed weight and is crucial for preventing bone and muscle mass loss. This is why combining daily high-intensity, cardio, and aerobic exercises with the right amount of protein to build and maintain your muscles is important.

High-intensity exercises like weightlifting and high-intensity interval training (HIIT) workouts are essential for building muscle and increasing overall strength. These exercises stress your muscles, prompting them to adapt and grow stronger. On the other hand, cardio and aerobic exercises are important for improving your heart health and endurance. By combining these different types of exercises, you can enhance your overall physical fitness and achieve your weight loss and muscle gain goals even quicker.

I often do a high-intensity 45-minute or 1-hour workout on my elliptical the first thing in the morning, whether it's 35 degrees or 95 degrees outside. This helps ensure that I can get my daily exercise done. I found that the longer I wait to do it later in the day, the less likely I am to make it.

In addition, I still do at least 60 jumping jacks every 2–3 hours, 60 aerobic step jumps the next 2–3 hours or when I have a break or feel like I need movement throughout the day. I often use the resistance bands to stretch over my shoulder after every couple hours of working on the computer.

In addition to exercise, it's important to **fuel your body with the right amount of protein. Protein is the building block of muscles** and is necessary for repairing and rebuilding muscle tissue broken down during exercise. Without enough protein, your muscles may not recover properly, hindering your progress in building muscle mass. Incorporating high-quality lean protein sources into your meals during your eating windows, such as lean meats, wild fish, eggs, and plant-based sources like quinoa, lentils, and tofu will support your muscle-building goals.

By combining daily exercise with the right amount of lean protein, you can achieve your weight loss and muscle gain goals and improve your overall health and well-being. Remember to listen to your body and give it the rest and recovery it needs, as overtraining can lead to injury and hinder your progress, but do your best not to skip it when you have time.

With dedication, consistency, and the right approach, you can achieve a strong, healthy, and toned body that you can be proud of.

Setting achievable fitness goals and staying with the exercise you enjoy most is crucial to keep you motivated and focused on increasing physical activity. Whether it's being able to run a certain distance daily, doing a certain number of push-ups every day, or doing one hour or more of cardio so that you can reach your specific health and/or weight goal, having something to work toward with commitments gives you the motivation to stay consistent with your workouts.

You can also find a workout buddy or join a fitness class to stay accountable and motivated to exercise regularly. Having someone to exercise with can make the experience more enjoyable and help keep you on track with your fitness journey.

Finally, as your fitness level improves, gradually increase the intensity and duration of your workouts. This progression is essential for continuous improvement and ensuring that your body continues to be challenged for better and lasting health benefits.

Here's How I Do It

I get in a scheduled workout each day in the morning, before noon. If my schedule doesn't allow me to work out before noon, I will do it before dinner. I don't want to work out three to four hours before bedtime. This is important because exercising too close to bedtime interferes with sleep.

I often only do at least two to three exercises out of all of the suggested exercises below daily.

1. **Elliptical** – 30 minutes to 1 hour a day at intensity level 10 to 15

2. **Aerobic step jumps** – 30 easy jumps up to 6 times a day

3. 20–30 **squats** 6 times/day, whether you're in your office or at home

4. 30–60 **jumping jacks** 6 times/day

5. **Resistance bands** – I stretch the band over my shoulder – 30 stretches 4 – 6 times/day to help with neck or shoulder pain

6. **Hand weights or dumbbells** – I lift with a 2lbs or a 5-lb dumbbell on each hand with 30 lifts 2–4 times/day

7. I use **a fitness tracker and a smart scale** to monitor my progress and keep me motivated to reach my fitness goals

8. I use **a workout planner and journal** to help my schedule and track my

workouts, keeping me organized and committed to my fitness goals

My favorite way of keeping myself on track to finish my daily workout on the elliptical is by listening to my favorite audiobooks, new course(s) with available audio versions, or new playlists of all my favorite songs.

LEVEL UP YOUR WORKOUTS

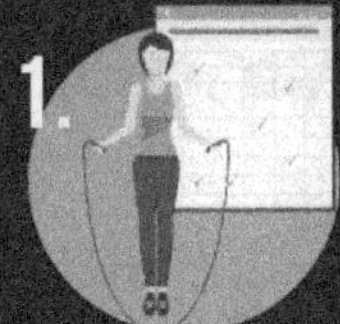

1. Create and schedule your daily workout sessions on your calendar and set reminders on your phone, commit to this daily exercise routine.

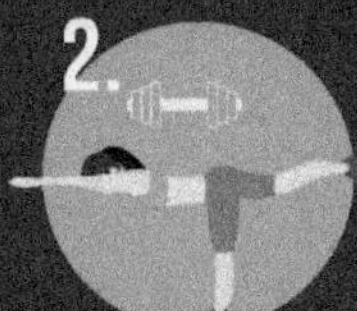

2. Incorporate a mix of cardio and strength training exercises into your daily exercise routine to maximize the benefits for your metabolism and weight loss goals.

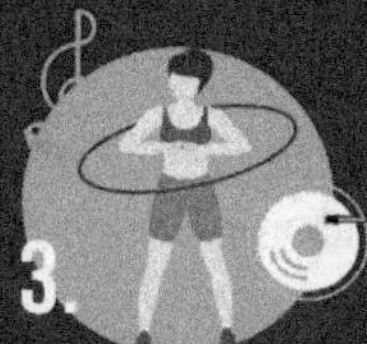

3. Create a playlist with your favorite songs or line up your favorite audio books to keep you motivated and focused on increasing physical activity.

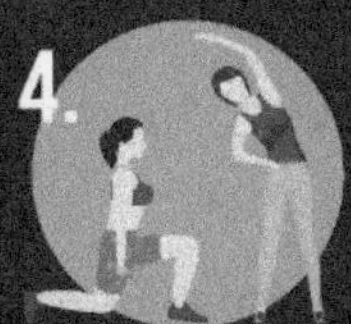

4. Find a workout buddy or join a fitness class to stay accountable and motivated to exercise regularly.

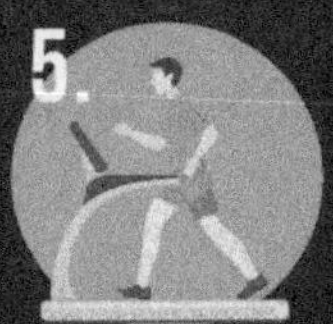

5. Increase the intensity and duration of your workouts to the level you feel comfortable with for better health improvement.

Chapter 5
Elite Eating: Choosing Nutrient-Dense Foods for Maximum Health Benefits

Welcome to Chapter 5 of *Fast, Lean, Strong*! In this chapter, we will discuss the importance of prioritizing nutrient-dense foods and how to create a meal plan that focuses on whole, nutrient-dense foods such as fruits, vegetables, lean proteins, and healthy fats.

This chapter will help you:

- Understand the importance of prioritizing whole, nutrient-dense foods for simultaneous sustained energy, better health, and weight loss

- Learn how to create a meal plan focusing on fruits, vegetables, lean proteins, and healthy fats to support your weight-loss goals

- Discover the significance of having the right protein daily and monitoring portion sizes to avoid overeating and support your weight loss journey

- Educate yourself on the nutritional content of different foods using resources like USDA FoodData Central and MyFitnessPal for informed choices

- Use the Continuous Glucose Monitoring (CGM) tool (if you have access to) daily to monitor calorie intake and your body's response to food

- Explore new and exciting ways to prepare nutrient-dense ingredients, keeping your meals interesting and delicious while prioritizing your health

How My Boyfriend's Severe Allergic Reaction Vanished through the Power of Whole Foods

It was a typical Wednesday when my boyfriend, Glen, came home from work. He was exhausted from a long day at the paper mill, where he had been working on software programming. As he walked through the door, I couldn't help but notice the redness and swelling around his eyes and his mouth. It was clear that something was seriously wrong.

He'd had a severe allergic reaction, and we were both at a loss as to what could have caused it. Could it have been the food he had for breakfast at work, or was it some chemical exposure in the factory? Glen had never experienced anything like this before.

With Covid restrictions in place, it was hard to know for sure, and we were left to wonder and worry.

His discomfort was evident, with a few painful blisters cropping up around his lips and mouth, making it difficult for him to eat. He was not fond of seeking medical attention, especially with the state of hospitals and medical facilities during the pandemic. It was a tough time for everyone, and we couldn't bear the thought of adding extra stress to an already chaotic situation.

I took it upon myself to research and find a solution. I scoured the internet, read e-books, and visited reputable health websites searching for home remedies and treatments that might offer relief. While most of the advice I found recommended seeking professional healthcare advice for severe symptoms, I was determined to do whatever I could with the resources available to me. I knew I had to take action to help Glen feel better soon. Thankfully, he's a very positive person, which also helped tremendously.

I set to work, carefully shopping and selecting a variety of lean proteins of beef, salmon, and chicken, and fresh, natural green vegetables, mushrooms, and fresh herbs to prepare different meals, mainly soups.

These nourishing, wholesome meals provided much-needed relief for Glen with their natural vitamins and minerals that improved his immunity first and foremost. He also has high-quality, hot herbal teas throughout the day, every day.

After two full days of sticking to those meals, drinks, and rests, we were both amazed that the redness and swelling had significantly decreased and the blisters were beginning to fade. It was an emotional moment for both of us as tears of joy and relief filled our eyes. It seemed that the power of whole, fresh foods had worked wonders for Glen's condition, and we were grateful for their positive impact.

By the fourth day, the blisters and redness had vanished entirely, and Glen felt like himself again. It was a remarkable transformation, and it had all been achieved without medication. He hadn't even reached for an Advil or ibuprofen to ease his discomfort because he's the type of guy who doesn't want to depend on any medication. Instead, his optimism and the healing power of nutritious, wholesome foods turned things around for him.

We also found that Glen had lost over seven pounds as an unexpected yet welcome bonus. It was a testament to our positive changes in his diet, choosing fresh and whole foods over processed, canned, or frozen options, like when he lived alone, or over mainly fried and fast foods with his co-workers during work. It was a profound realization that our bodies respond to our choices, and when we choose wisely, the rewards can be transformative.

Ultimately, this experience reminded us that **our bodies have incredible healing capabilities. Still, it's up to us to provide them with the right quality nourishment and care**. Regarding our health, proactive and positive actions are key to achieving our goals. We learned that making healthy choices is not just about hoping for the best and waiting for things to improve; it's about taking intentional steps, **making wise decisions on quality healthy food and drink choices**, and allowing our bodies to do what they do best – heal and thrive.

Glen's recovery was a powerful testament to the impact of healthy, whole-food choices, and it served as a profound lesson for both of us. We celebrated that we had taken control of his health in a tumultuous time and had experienced firsthand **the remarkable impact of embracing nutritious, nourishing, whole foods**. It was a transformative journey that brought us closer together and left us with a newfound appreciation for the healing power of whole foods and the positive actions we can take to improve our health.

Use the table below to calculate your right daily needed protein amount.

HAVE LEAN PROTEIN DAILY TO BUILD HEALTHY MUSCLE!

Protein basic calculation:

Lean protein such as
beef, salmon, chicken

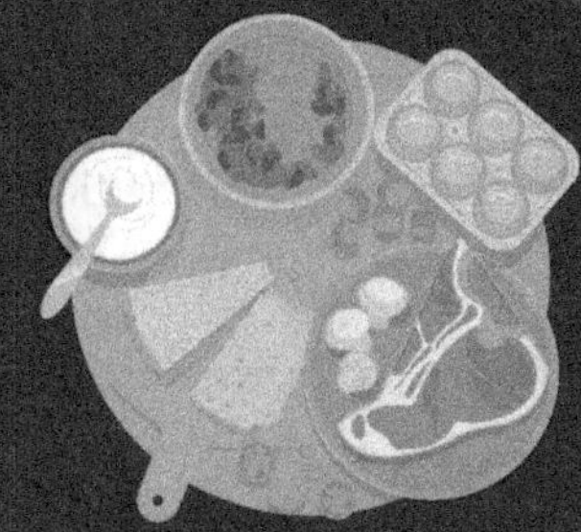

Total weight of the food g × Percentage of protein in the food = Protein g

For example, if a food item weighs 200g (7 oz.) and contains 40% protein, the calculation would be:
Protein g = 200g (7 oz.) × 0.40 = 80g (2.8 oz.)

Daily Protein Intake Amount Recommendation:

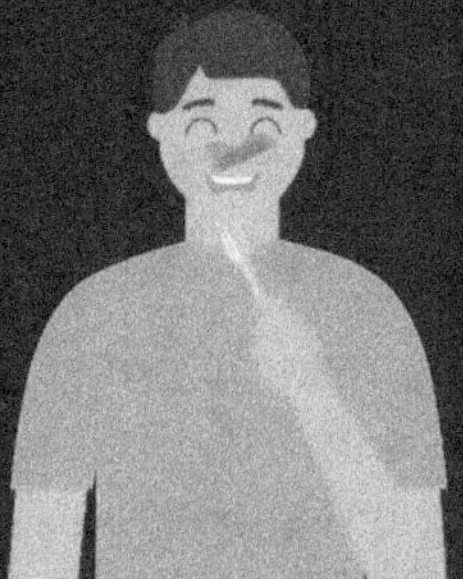

2g protein x per Kg body weight per day.
(Convert Lbs. to Kg and convert g to oz.)

For example, I weight 120 Lbs.
So 2g x 54.4 kg = 108.8g (3.8oz.) of protein a day

Possible Tools and Resources You Will Need

- Your phone's Notes

- Meal planning apps: Mealime, Noom

- Nutritional information databases: USDA FoodData Central, Mayo Clinic, WebMD, Harvard Health, British Heart Foundation, MyFitnessPal

- If you have access to the Continuous Glucose Monitoring (CGM) tool, then use it daily to monitor your body's response to food and to modify your nutrition plans

- Cooking books and recipes **focused on whole, fresh, anti-inflammatory, immunity foods**

- Meal prep containers

After your fasting windows end, the fresh and high-quality foods you consume are crucial in supporting your body's needs and providing sustained energy. It's especially important to ensure your meals are packed with fresh, natural, whole foods with nutrients, regardless of whether your goal is to achieve an ideal weight, better lasting health, or ideally both.

First, let's discuss creating a meal plan focused on whole, nutrient-dense foods. This means incorporating a variety of fruits, vegetables, lean proteins such as lean beef fillet, chicken, turkey, and fish, and healthy fats like wild salmon, avocados, nuts, and olive oil into your meals.

Daily protein intake (please use the table in the previous page to calculate your daily needed protein amount based on your body weight) **and daily exercise are essential to developing and maintaining muscle mass during intermittent fasting**.

Consuming the right amount of protein daily provides the building blocks for muscle growth and repair. The combination of daily protein intake and exercise helps increase muscle protein synthesis, leading to the development and maintenance of muscle mass.

Without enough protein and exercise, the body may struggle to retain or build muscle, potentially losing strength and muscle mass over time.

Furthermore, adequate lean protein intake and regular physical activity are important for muscle growth and maintenance and contribute to overall lasting health and well-being. Consuming enough lean protein can help support a healthy metabolism, regulate appetite, and optimize body composition.

In addition, engaging in regular exercise has numerous health benefits, including improved cardiovascular function, increased bone density, and reduced risk of chronic diseases. Thus, the combination of daily lean protein intake and daily exercise promotes muscle mass and provides lasting health benefits for individuals of all ages.

Another important step is to **monitor your meal portion sizes and protein amounts to avoid overeating** and to support your weight loss goals. It's crucial to be mindful of portion sizes when it comes time to eat.

After fasting for a while, it's easy to feel ravenous and want to indulge in large or excessive portions. However, this can counteract the benefits of the fasting period and lead to overconsumption of calories. Portion control is key to maintaining a healthy, balanced diet, especially with intermittent fasting.

Controlling your daily meal and snack sizes can help you better manage your hunger and **prevent excessive calorie intake**. It's important to listen to your body's hunger cues and **stop eating when you feel satisfied** rather than uncomfortably full. You can **meet your body's nutritional needs** by **controlling** your **portion sizes without overdoing it**.

Consuming large portions of food after fasting can also lead to rapid spikes in blood sugar, which can harm your overall health. You can maintain more stable blood sugar levels by controlling your portion sizes.

So, **remember to be mindful of portion sizes and listen to your body's cues to prevent overconsumption after your fasting hours.**

Additionally, it's essential to learn the nutritional content of different foods to make informed, healthy food choices. Utilize resources like the USDA FoodData Central and MyFitnessPal to identify the nutrient content of your consumed foods. This knowledge, together with the suggested daily protein intake (please use the protein calculation table in this chapter) will empower you to make healthier food choices with the right amount to ensure you get the essential vitamins and minerals your body needs from those wholesome foods.

Plan your meals ahead to ensure you have solid healthy food options during your eating windows. This will help you avoid reaching for processed or unhealthy foods when you're hungry.

If you have access to the Continuous Glucose Monitoring (CGM) tool, use it daily to monitor your body's response to food, and modify your meal plans accordingly to ensure you are adequately nourished, not under or over.

Lastly, seek new and exciting ways to prepare nutrient-dense ingredients to keep your meals interesting. Explore cooking and recipe books focused on healthy, whole foods to discover delicious and creative recipes that prioritize nutrient-dense ingredients.

Infuse Flavor and Nutrition into Post-Fasting Meals with Nutrient-Dense Ingredients

Explore new and exciting ways to cook and prepare your meals:

1. Experiment with different cooking methods: Try steaming, grilling with indoor grills, and sautéing nutrient-dense ingredients such as leafy green vegetables, mushrooms, lean proteins (chicken, fish, lean fillet red meats, tofu), and non-starchy root vegetables (or remove the starch with the 7-hour soaking in the <u>Note</u> below) to keep your meals exciting and nutritious.

   <u>Note</u>: **slightly undercook your green veggies and mushrooms to preserve their nutrition**. If you want **to remove starch** from root veggies such as white potatoes, peel the potato skin off, cut them into quarter or chunk sizes, and **soak them in water for seven to eight hours** before cooking. You can also soak the white rice this way to reduce the starch content.

2. Incorporate **superfoods of leafy greens and mushrooms** into your everyday meals: Seek out nutrient-dense superfoods of all leafy green veggies like **kale, broccolini, Brussels sprouts**, then **lentils, quinoa, chia seeds, and berries** to add a boost of natural vitamins, minerals, and antioxidants to your meals after your intermittent fasting window.

3. Explore global cuisines: Look into recipes from different cultures that focus on nutrient-dense ingredients such as **chicken or beef lentils with carrot soups from Europe, Japanese sushi and grilled fish** style, **smoked fish**, and seaweed, or **Mediterranean salads with olive oil, nuts, leafy greens, and fresh herbs** to keep your meals exciting and diverse.

4. Get creative with meal prepping: Experiment with whole, fresh, nutrient-dense ingredients by preparing colorful and flavorful salads, nourishing grain bowls, and satisfying homemade soups with fresh ingredients to keep your meals interesting throughout the week. Strategically, **every daily meal** of

yours **should have at least <u>three colors of natural whole foods</u>** – for example, sautéed **green beans**, roasted or grilled **chicken breast**, and roasted **orange sweet potatoes**. Another example will be roasted brussels sprouts,

5. Utilize fresh herbs and spices: Enhance not only the flavor of your nutrient-dense ingredients but also the attractive look of your meals by using a variety of fresh herbs and spices such as rosemary, sweet basil, ginger, cinnamon, nutmeg, turmeric, and cumin to add depth and complexity to your meals after your intermittent fasting windows.

<u>It's time to say goodbye to canned, processed, and fried foods</u> (including fries and chips) and hello to more delicious, nourishing meals with **fresh, green, whole foods** that **so essential to improve not only your immunity but also your metabolic health.**

To simplify your journey, consider using meal planning apps like Mealime or Noom to streamline the meal planning process. These apps can help you organize your meals, generate grocery lists, calculate protein amounts, and discover new recipes based on your dietary preferences. Or you can simply just use your own phone's Notes to record all of the above for easier and quicker access. I still do that 100%.

In conclusion, prioritizing nutrient-dense foods is key to supporting your body's needs, boosting metabolism, and achieving your health and weight-loss goals. Remember to add your daily right amount of lean protein to your post-fast meals too to ensure your muscle gain. This is true even if you're not doing intermittent fasting. But if you are, adding these awesome eats into your daily meals after your fasting windows can help you achieve your goals way quicker!

Don't forget to do at least 2 of the simple exercise movements in chapter 4 every day. Your body will thank you!

By creating a meal plan focused on whole, fresh, nutrient-dense foods, preparing your meals in advance, monitoring portion sizes, and educating yourself on nutritional content, you can ensure your body receives the essential nutrients needed to thrive.

So, let's start cooking and nourishing your body with the best foods for a healthier you!

POST-FASTING
EATING WINDOWS CHEKLIST

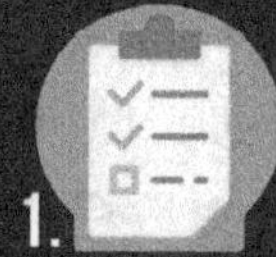

- [ ] Write down a list of whole, nutrient-dense foods that you will commit to get for your grocery shopping list, to cook at home, or to keep in the back of your mind when you eat out.

1.

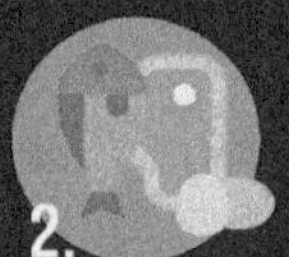

2.

- [ ] Create a meal plan that focuses on fruits, vegetables, lean proteins, and healthy fats (avocados, wild salmon...) to support your health and your weight loss goals.

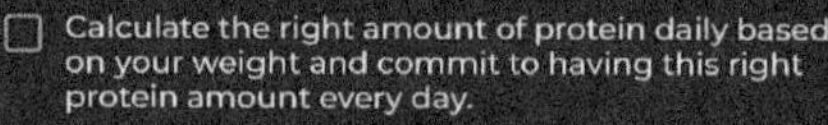

- [ ] Calculate the right amount of protein daily based on your weight and commit to having this right protein amount every day.

3.

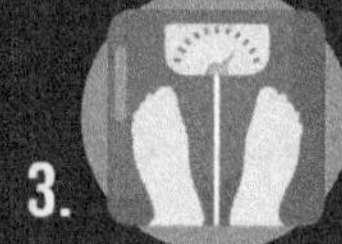

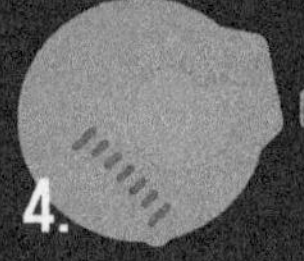

4.

- [ ] Pay attention to nutritional content on food labels for informed choices on reducing added sugar and fat during your eating windows.

- [ ] Explore new ways to have or to prepare meals with only nutrient-dense ingredients, keeping your meals interesting and delicious while prioritizing your health.

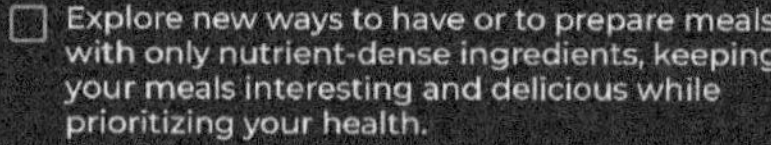

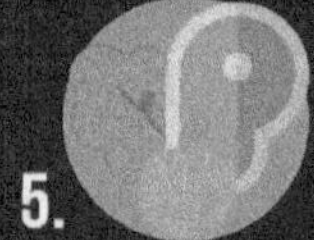

5.

- [ ] Use the Continuous Glucose Monitoring (CGM) tool daily (if you have access to the tool) to monitor calorie intake and food response to your body.

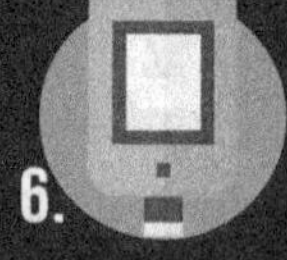

6.

Chapter 6
The Power of Tracking to Maintain IF Practice Daily or Weekly: Identifying Triggers and Habits to Supercharge Your Intermittent Fasting Results

In this chapter, we will explore the importance of keeping a detailed diary/journal of your fasting and exercise schedules, fasting drinks, and eating habits.

In addition, this chapter will help you:

- Create a detailed diary/journal to track your fasting schedule, food intake, and energy levels, allowing you to identify patterns and make necessary adjustments

- Utilize food-tracking apps like Mealime or your phone's Notes to monitor and keep track of your calorie intake and macronutrient balance, providing valuable insights into your eating habits and aiding in informed decision-making

- Reflect on your eating patterns to identify consistent habits or triggers that may affect your fasting progress, enabling you to work on changing them and improving your results

- Analyze your gathered data to determine your most effective fasting style and schedule, adjusting your eating patterns based on the information

- Gain valuable insights into what works best for your body and lifestyle, making necessary changes to achieve your health and fitness goals

How I Mastered the Art of Self-Control with Consistent Intermittent Fasting (IF) Practice and Transformed My Life – and How You Can Too!

Sitting here at my desk, penning this final chapter, I can't help but reflect on the woman in the blue dress in tears back in 2016. Fast forward to today, and I can confidently say that I've never struggled with my weight since then. I've always had it under control.

Let me paint a picture of my life now: I don't stress about gaining a few pounds because I know I can always bounce back. I'm really not some ascetic monk subsisting on a diet of sawdust and soy milk. I've just mastered the art of self-control with intermittent fasting (IF), and the confidence and empowerment that come with it are invaluable.

And it's not just about me. If you've ever been able to help someone in your own journey, you'll understand the profound impact this can have.

These days, intermittent fasting has given me the gift of not having to worry about my weight, not having the neck pain, feeling out of breath and many other benefits. I want nothing more than for you to experience the same remarkable results. I encourage you to start practicing intermittent fasting (IF) as soon as you can to unlock the potential for greatness in your own life.

These simple IF practices I use daily are important because they keep me on track!

- Mark the fasting timeframe and exercise time on your calendar and set reminders on your phone for each day.

- Set specific times for having your fasting drinks to the specific hours for each day on your phone according to your work, commute, and family times.

- Set in advance specific meal plans with lean protein, whole foods, and fresh nutrition for each meal of each day.

- Clear your pantry, fridge, and counter areas of snacks, foods, and drinks that might make you break your fasting.

- Wait, did you start eating a bit too soon? No sweat – just get back on track with your fasting plan the next day. But keep in mind, the more slips you have, the longer it might take to hit your health and weight loss targets.

The steps I'm sharing below are extra crucial for understanding what works best for you to maximize your intermittent fasting results and to maintain your IF practices consistently so that you can do it daily, every other day, weekly, or a combination.

Step 1: Utilize a journal or use your phone's Notes

Use a notebook or just open up the Notes app on your phone and start jotting down everything, every hour if you can, from what you want and need, to what you like and dislike. Write about what's working and what's not from day one. Then, the next day, take a look at your notes, see what's up, and tweak things as needed.

Keep up with this note-taking every day—it's a cool habit that'll help you stay on track with your fasting times.

You can also use one of the food-tracking apps that I mentioned earlier to monitor your calorie intake and macronutrient balance. This can help you meet your nutritional needs during your eating window and prevent overeating.

Step 2: Reflect on your eating patterns

Remember to take the time to reflect on your eating patterns and identify any consistent habits or triggers affecting your fasting progress. For example, do you tend to reach for snacks when stressed, or do you mindlessly eat in front of your computer, the TV, on your phone, or when you drive?

Recognizing these patterns can help you make strategic changes to support your fasting goals. But if you don't record as in Step 1 and don't reflect as in Step 2, you might forget and fall into the same patterns the next day. As a result, they might stop you or slow you down from achieving your health and weight loss goals.

Step 3: Seek support when you need it most

If you find that emotional or stress-related eating habits are impacting your progress, don't hesitate to seek support. Consider seeking an intermittent fasting accountability partner, a great friend who you know can help you, or a community with members who can share with you about successful IF practices.

You can also contact a nutritionist or counselor who can help you analyze and address these habits, providing valuable tools and strategies to manage them effectively.

Step 4: Analyze Your Results

After experimenting with different fasting schedules and keeping a journal, take the time to analyze your results. Look for patterns in how your body responds to each fasting style. Identify the schedules that align with your lifestyle and schedules that produce the best results in curbing your appetite, reducing hunger cravings, keeping you up with having exercise then healthy meals. By doing so, you'll be able to determine your most effective fasting style and schedule. Again, check for my journal examples in Chapter 2 and in this Chapter, under How do I do this.

Adjust your eating patterns

Use the insights from tracking and analyzing your food choices and habits to adjust your eating patterns. Whether tasting different fasting drinks, choosing more healthy satiating foods, finding alternative coping mechanisms for stress, or reevaluating your fasting schedule in whole, making targeted adjustments as soon as you can, can significantly enhance your intermittent fasting experience and give you the result quicker.

Resources and Tools

- Your favorite notebook, journal, color markers, calendar, and your phone

You can use the old-fashion notebook or journal to record all activities before, during, and after your fasting hours. You can also mark your fasting schedules on your calendar then your phone's reminder again for extra useful help.

Or consider using digital food diaries or meal-tracking apps for convenience and accuracy in tracking your eating patterns. You just need to download and sign up for those apps. There are also mood and emotion-tracking apps or journals that can help you monitor and address emotional or stress-related eating habits.

How do I do this?

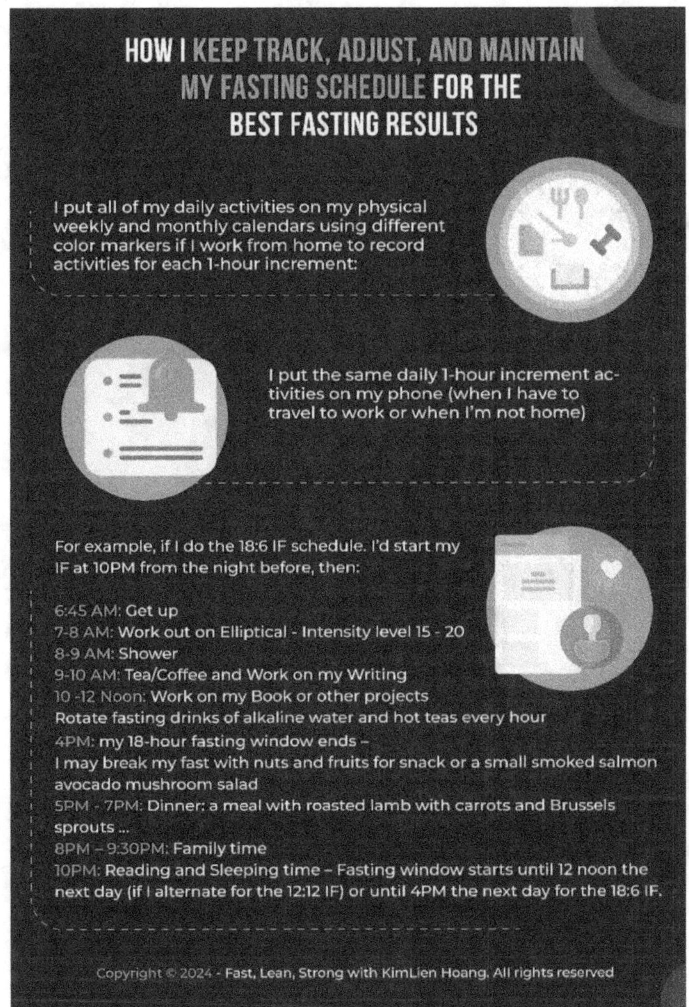

I put all of my daily activities on my weekly and monthly calendars, including my fasting schedules and eating windows since each day's schedule of mine might be slightly different than the next.

I use different marker colors to mark working, fasting, eating, travel, and unexpected changes.

I put on my phone schedule what to shop and/or cook for each day during my eating windows. I even note the times I eat out.

Don't forget, you can seek out online support groups or forums tailored to individuals practicing intermittent fasting for guidance and insight.

Lastly, utilize resources such as self-help books or health websites to address emotional and stress-related eating habits, empowering you to make positive changes.

By implementing these steps and utilizing the suggested resources, you can effectively track and analyze your fasting and eating habits, ultimately supercharging your intermittent fasting results and achieving your health and weight-loss goals

Checklist for Your Action Steps

- ✓ Create a detailed diary/journal to track your fasting schedule, food intake, and energy levels, allowing you to identify patterns and make necessary adjustments.

- ✓ Download a minimum of one food-tracking app or use the CGM tool or your Notes to monitor your calorie intake and macronutrient balance, providing valuable insights into your eating habits and aiding in informed decision-making.

- ✓ Identify consistent habits or triggers in your diary/journal that may affect your fasting progress; work on changing them and improving your results.

- ✓ Analyze the gathered data from your diary/journal to determine your most effective fasting style and schedule, and adjust your eating patterns based on the identified patterns to achieve your health and fitness goals.

Conclusion

Congratulations on finishing *Fast, Lean, Strong: A Simple Five-Step Guide to Master Intermittent Fasting (IF) for Weight Loss, Muscle Gain, and for Lasting Health Benefits*! You are now armed with the knowledge and practical advice to truly succeed in your intermittent fasting journey.

Whether you're an IF beginner or you may have struggled with IF in the past, you now have the power to change the game and achieve your weight loss, muscle-building, and overall health goals.

The strategies and tips outlined in the book are designed to help you overcome the common hurdles of intermittent fasting, such as feeling starved, experiencing food cravings, and dealing with fatigue during fasting windows.

By implementing the practical advice and examples, you can create an effective intermittent fasting plan that works for you, your body, your work schedule, and your lifestyle.

<u>It's time to take action.</u>

Write down your IF goals and actions to achieve each goal NOW.

<u>Your first step</u> is to set some **specific goals** and develop the mindset to commit to them to achieve great results with IF.

Identify one to three specific goals that you want to achieve with IF, such as:

1. losing a certain amount of weight
2. increasing your energy levels
3. improving your metabolic or overall health

What are you specific IF success goals?

<u>Second step</u>, set a realistic timeline for X number of days or weeks for achieving these goals, and then envision the amazing results you will achieve once you reach them with IF.

To make your goals a reality, you need to take specific actions.

For example,

- Clear out your pantry of unhealthy snacks and processed foods
- Stock up on the right fasting drinks that will support your IF hours
- Create a weekly meal plan with only whole, nutrient-dense, fresh foods

Next, **pick your intermittent fasting (IF) hours** for your specific days or the whole first week, **mark them on your calendar, and schedule them on your phone to start your IF immediately**.

Whether you choose a 12:12 IF and alternate with 18:6 IF daily or combine with One Meal a Day or any other fasting style, test then commit to them and stick with them.

Remember, **the key to IF success** lies in **consistency**.

Once you have established your fasting schedule, it's important to follow through with the other four steps outlined in the book. This includes:

1. Keeping up with only fasting drinks through your fasting hours
2. Fueling your body with the proper nutrients during your eating window
3. Incorporating daily exercise (even just 30 minutes, but 45 minutes or longer will help your body much more), and
4. Maintaining your new working IF practices daily or weekly.

By **following each step diligently and practicing IF correctly and persistently**, you will **soon see positive changes in your body** and overall well-being.

Sometimes, intermittent fasting may seem daunting, especially when the cravings kick in, so always consider the difference between hunger and cravings. With discipline, determination for better health, and a solid IF plan in place, you can transform your health and achieve your desired results.

Stay committed, stay motivated, and most importantly, **believe in yourself**.

Remember, you are not alone in this journey. Connect with others, practice intermittent fasting, seek support, and, most importantly, be patient with yourself. Your body will adapt to the new eating and fasting routine, and the results will soon follow.

So, what are you waiting for? It's time to take the first step toward a healthier, leaner, and stronger you. Implement the knowledge you have gained from this book and **start your intermittent fasting journey today**.

It's time to get results!

Introducing KimLien Hoang, the Ultimate Intermittent Fasting Contriver

As a family woman and dedicated mom to my amazing son, I understand the struggle of balancing a hectic schedule while prioritizing health and fitness. After successfully achieving my ideal body weight and shedding over 9lbs in less than 12 days through intermittent fasting (IF), I was inspired to share my IF journey and knowledge with those who want to start IF and who may be struggling to reach your weight loss and fitness goals with IF.

I wrote this book to share a simple yet effective five-step guide to mastering intermittent fasting for weight loss, muscle gain, and lasting health benefits after my own trials, errors, and wins. I want to empower beginners and struggling intermittent fasters with the strategies you need to overcome plateaus and incorporate daily exercise into your fasting routine. My goal is to help you achieve your weight loss goals and improve your overall fitness with confidence through intermittent fasting.

As an herbal and nutrition research enthusiast, a lover of tea and coffee, a devoted cook, and an admirer of golf and travel, I bring a unique and diverse perspective to intermittent fasting. My passion for health and wellness drives me to constantly seek new and innovative ways to help people achieve their fitness and weight loss goals.

So, if you're ready to take charge of your health and start seeing actual results, I urge you to read *Fast, Lean, Strong: A Simple Five-Step Guide to Mastering Intermittent Fasting (IF)* right now. Together, we can embark on the IF journey the simple way toward a healthier, happier, and more confident YOU.

Let's Make Your Intermittent Fasting Practice the Change Worth Doing!

Glossary Definitions

Blood Sugar Levels: *The measurement of glucose in the blood.* Intermittent fasters need to understand how their eating habits and exercise impact their blood sugar levels to manage energy levels and hunger throughout the fasting period.

Caloric Deficit: *When the amount of calories consumed is less than the amount of calories burned.* Intermittent fasters aiming for weight loss must maintain a caloric deficit to achieve their goals.

Carb Cycling: *A dietary approach alternating between high and low carbohydrate intake.* This can be utilized by intermittent fasters to optimize energy levels and fat loss during their fasting period.

Eating Window: *The specific timeframe in which an individual consumes their meals during intermittent fasting.* Understanding and sticking to an eating window is crucial for achieving weight loss and fitness goals.

Fat Adaptation: *The body's transition to using fat as its primary fuel source, commonly experienced during intermittent fasting.* Intermittent fasters need to become fat-adapted to maximize fat loss and energy levels.

Fasting Endurance: *The ability to sustain longer fasting periods without experiencing extreme hunger or adverse side effects.* Building fasting endurance is crucial for intermittent fasters to stick to their fasting schedule and achieve their weight-loss goals.

High-Intensity Interval Training (HIIT): *A form of exercise that alternates between short, intense bursts of activity and periods of recovery.* HIIT benefits intermittent fasters by enhancing fat burning and improving overall fitness within a limited workout time.

Insulin Sensitivity: *The body can efficiently process glucose and regulate blood sugar levels.* Insulin sensitivity is essential for intermittent fasters to optimize fat loss and metabolic health.

Ketogenic Diet: *A high-fat, moderate-protein, low-carbohydrate diet that can be paired with intermittent fasting to enhance fat burning and promote weight loss.*

Meal Timing: *The specific timing of meals within the eating window during* *intermittent fasting.* Proper meal timing can impact energy levels, hunger, and overall success in achieving fitness and weight-loss goals.

Metabolism: *The process by which the body converts food and drink into energy.* Understanding and optimizing metabolism is important for intermittent fasters to maximize fat loss and overall fitness.

Muscle Recovery: *The process by which the muscles repair and grow stronger after exercise.* Proper muscle recovery is essential for intermittent fasters to optimize their workout performance and achieve fitness goals.

Plateau: *A state of little or no change in weight loss or fitness progress.* Overcoming plateaus is a common challenge for intermittent fasters, requiring strategic adjustments in diet and exercise.

Resistance Training: *An exercise involving resistance to induce muscular contractions, such as weightlifting or bodyweight exercises.* Resistance training is essential for intermittent fasters to preserve muscle mass and enhance fat loss.

Rest Days: *Scheduled days of rest from intense exercise.* Regular rest days are important for intermittent fasters to prevent burnout and promote recovery.

Strength Training: *Physical activity focused on improving muscular strength and endurance.* Incorporating strength training is crucial for intermittent fasters to preserve and build muscle mass and support fat loss.

Stalling: *A period of little to no progress in weight loss or fitness goals.* Overcoming stalling is a challenge for many intermittent fasters and requires strategic adjustments to diet and exercise.

Water Intake: *The amount of water consumed throughout the day.* Proper hydration is crucial for intermittent fasters to manage hunger and support metabolism and overall health.

Workout Frequency: *The number of workout sessions completed within a given timeframe.* Balancing workout frequency is crucial for intermittent fasters to promote muscle growth, fat loss, and overall fitness.

Portion Control: *Managing the food consumed at each meal or snack.* Practicing portion control is important for intermittent fasters to manage calorie intake and support weight loss goals.

Metabolic Flexibility: *The ability of the body to efficiently switch between using different fuel sources, such as carbohydrates and fats.* Developing metabolic flexibility is important for intermittent fasters to optimize fat burning and overall metabolic health.

Adherence: *The act of sticking to a plan or following guidelines.* Maintaining adherence to intermittent fasting and fitness strategies is essential for achieving weight-loss and fitness goals.

Calorie Cycling: *Alternating between higher and lower calorie intake on different days.* Intermittent fasters can utilize calorie cycling to prevent metabolic adaptation and enhance fat loss.

Nutrient Timing: *The strategic timing of nutrient intake, such as carbohydrates and protein, to support exercise performance and recovery.* Understanding nutrient timing is important for intermittent fasters to maximize the benefits of their workouts during fasting periods.

Hydration: *The process of consuming adequate fluids to maintain proper bodily functions.* Proper hydration is important for intermittent fasting to manage hunger, support metabolism, and improve overall health.

Stress Management: *Implementing techniques to reduce and cope with stress.* Effective stress management is important for intermittent fasters to optimize their mental and physical well-being, which can impact weight loss and fitness.

Mindful Eating: *The practice of being present and attentive while eating, focusing on the sensory experience and hunger cues.* Practicing mindful eating is important for intermittent fasters to manage portion control and prevent overeating during the eating window.

Progress Tracking: *Monitoring and assessing changes in weight, body composition, performance, and other fitness-related metrics.* Tracking progress is important for intermittent fasters to gauge the effectiveness of their strategies and make necessary adjustments.

Professional Guidance: *Seeking assistance from qualified experts such as nutritionists, personal trainers, or health coaches.* Professional guidance can help intermittent fasters optimize their strategies and overcome challenges in achieving weight-loss and fitness goals.

Positive Mindset: *A mental attitude focused on optimism, resilience, and confidence.* Cultivating a positive mindset is important for intermittent fasters to stay motivated, overcome challenges, and achieve long-term success.

Habit Formation: *The process of developing and maintaining consistent behaviors* *over time.* Establishing weekly intermittent fasting schedules with healthy habits is crucial for intermittent fasters to sustain their fasting, healthy nutrition, and fitness strategies, leading to long-term weight and health goals success.

15 Essential Answers to Overcoming Plateaus and Maximizing Your Intermittent Fasting Results

1. What is intermittent fasting and how does it contribute to weight loss?

Intermittent fasting is a pattern of eating that involves cycling between periods of eating and fasting. This can aid in weight loss by reducing overall calorie intake and increasing the body's ability to burn fat for fuel.

2. What are some common plateaus people experience with intermittent fasting?

Common plateaus with intermittent fasting include weight loss stagnation, decreased energy levels, and a slowed metabolism.

3. How can I overcome a plateau in intermittent fasting?

To overcome a plateau in intermittent fasting, you can try increasing your fasting window, picking the right fasting drinks, adjusting your meal timing, incorporating more low-carb, high-protein foods, and adding more physical activity.

4. What role does nutrition play in intermittent fasting and overcoming plateaus?

Nutrition plays a critical role in intermittent fasting and overcoming plateaus, as the types of foods you consume can influence your body's ability to burn fat and maintain energy levels.

5. How can I adjust my nutrition to support intermittent fasting and overcome plateaus?

To support intermittent fasting and overcome plateaus, you can focus on consuming whole, nutrient-dense foods, increasing your intake of healthy fats, and minimizing processed and high-sugar foods.

6. What are some effective daily exercise strategies to complement intermittent fasting for weight loss?

Incorporating regular exercise into your daily routine can help support weight loss and overcome plateaus. This can include a combination of aerobic exercise, strength training, and high-intensity interval training (HIIT).

7. Is it necessary to exercise while intermittent fasting?

Regular physical activity can enhance the weight loss benefits of fasting, improve muscle and lean mass, and promote overall health and wellness.

8. How can I adjust my exercise routine to overcome plateaus while intermittent fasting?

To overcome plateaus while intermittent fasting, you can adjust your exercise routine by increasing the intensity or duration of your workouts, incorporating new forms of exercise, and focusing on strength training to build muscle and boost metabolism.

9. What are some common mistakes people make when overcoming intermittent fasting plateaus?

Common mistakes people make when attempting to overcome intermittent fasting plateaus include not adjusting their fasting schedule, overeating and relying too heavily on processed or high-sugar foods, and neglecting regular physical activity.

10. How can I stay motivated to continue my intermittent fasting and exercise routine?

Staying motivated to stick with intermittent fasting and your exercise routine can be challenging. Still, you can stay focused by setting specific, achievable goals, finding a workout buddy for accountability, and rewarding yourself for meeting milestones.

11. Are there any specific supplements that support intermittent fasting and weight loss?

Some supplements, such as omega-3 fatty acids, vitamin D, and BCAAs, can support intermittent fasting and weight loss by promoting fat-burning, muscle recovery, and overall health.

12. How can I incorporate mindfulness and stress reduction into my intermittent fasting and exercise routine?

Incorporating mindfulness practices, such as meditation and deep breathing exercises, can help reduce stress levels, improve sleep quality, and support overall well-being while practicing intermittent fasting and exercising.

13. What are some long-term strategies for maintaining weight loss and optimal health after overcoming plateaus?

After overcoming plateaus, it's important to maintain a balanced, nutrient-dense diet, stay consistent with regular physical activity, and prioritize self-care and stress management.

14. Are any potential risks or side effects associated with long-term intermittent fasting (IF) and intense exercise?

Long-term intermittent fasting and intense exercise might pose potential risks, such as nutrient deficiencies, hormonal imbalances, and increased risk of injury if not practiced IF responsibly. It's very important to practice long-term IF with the right nutrition and the lean protein amount daily together with proper daily exercises and fitness guidance.

15. How can I seek professional guidance and support for my intermittent fasting and weight loss journey?

Seeking professional guidance and support from a registered dietitian, certified personal trainer, or healthcare provider can help you navigate your intermittent fasting and weight loss journey with tailored recommendations and personalized support.